Hambuggas
And
Frozen Peas

My Inspiration
This book is dedicated to, London and Lourde.

Heartfelt Thanks To

Natalya Kharitonova; *Illustrator*, for her amazing talent.

Kindle Direct Publishing
Seattle, WA 98108

Library of Congress Control Number 2019910011

ISBN: 9781723397646

Hambuggas

And

Frozen Peas

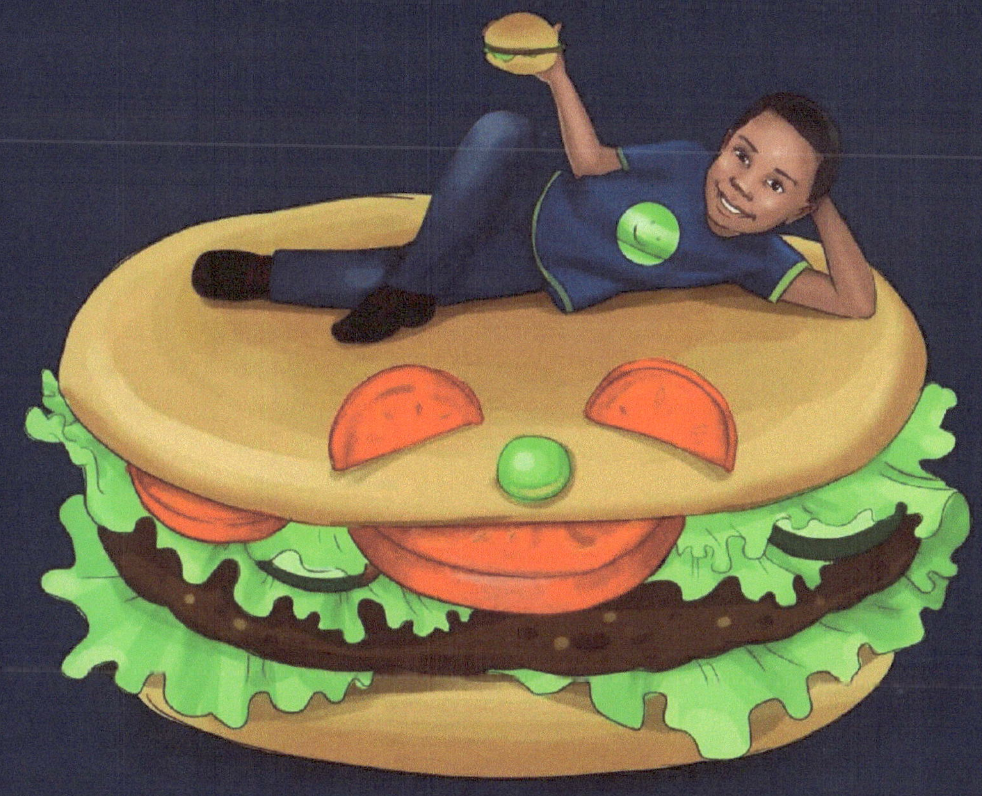

Author
Naejh

Illustrator
Natalya Kharitonova

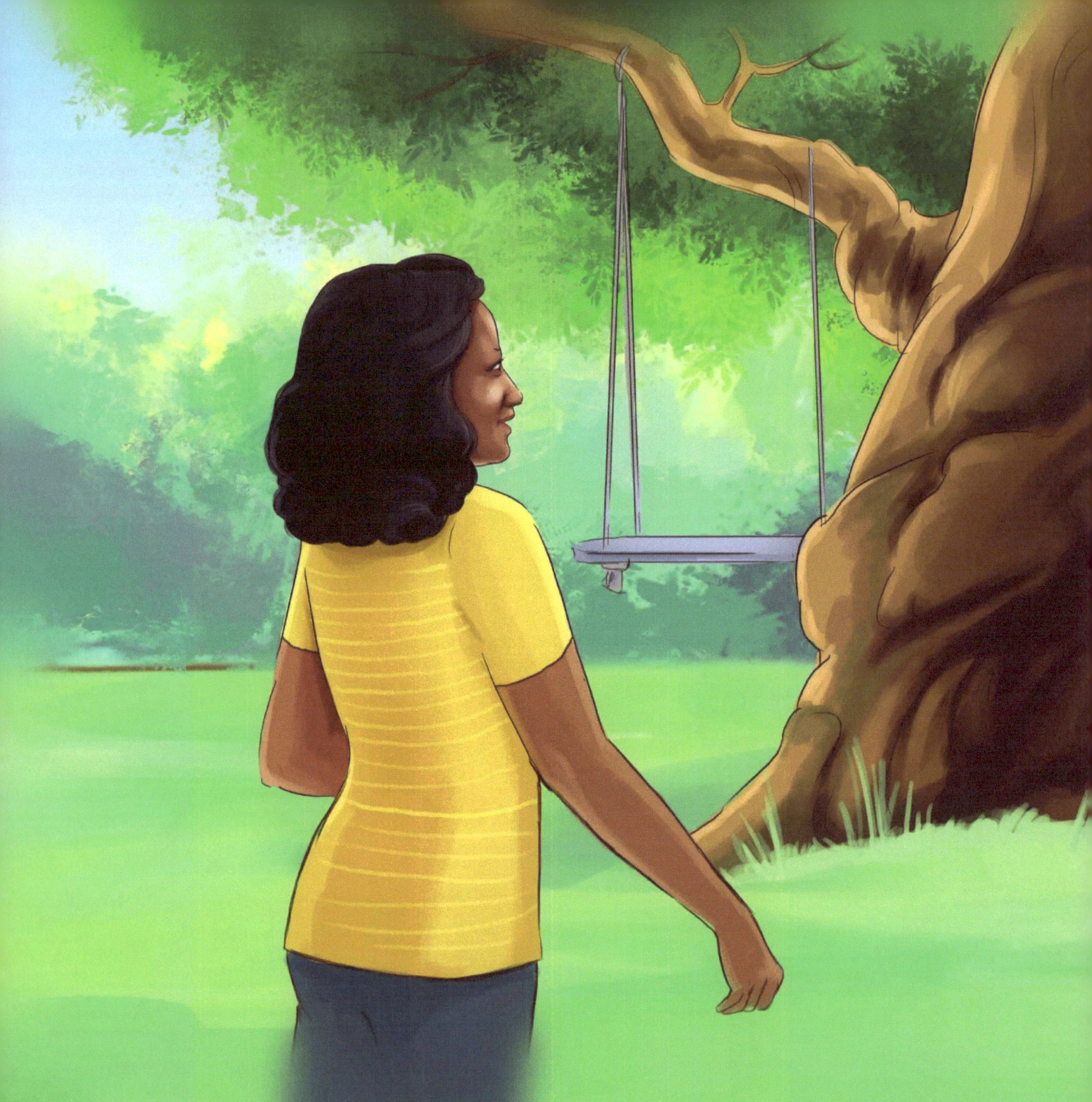

"Grandma asked, "Hey guys, it's lunch time, what do you want to eat?"

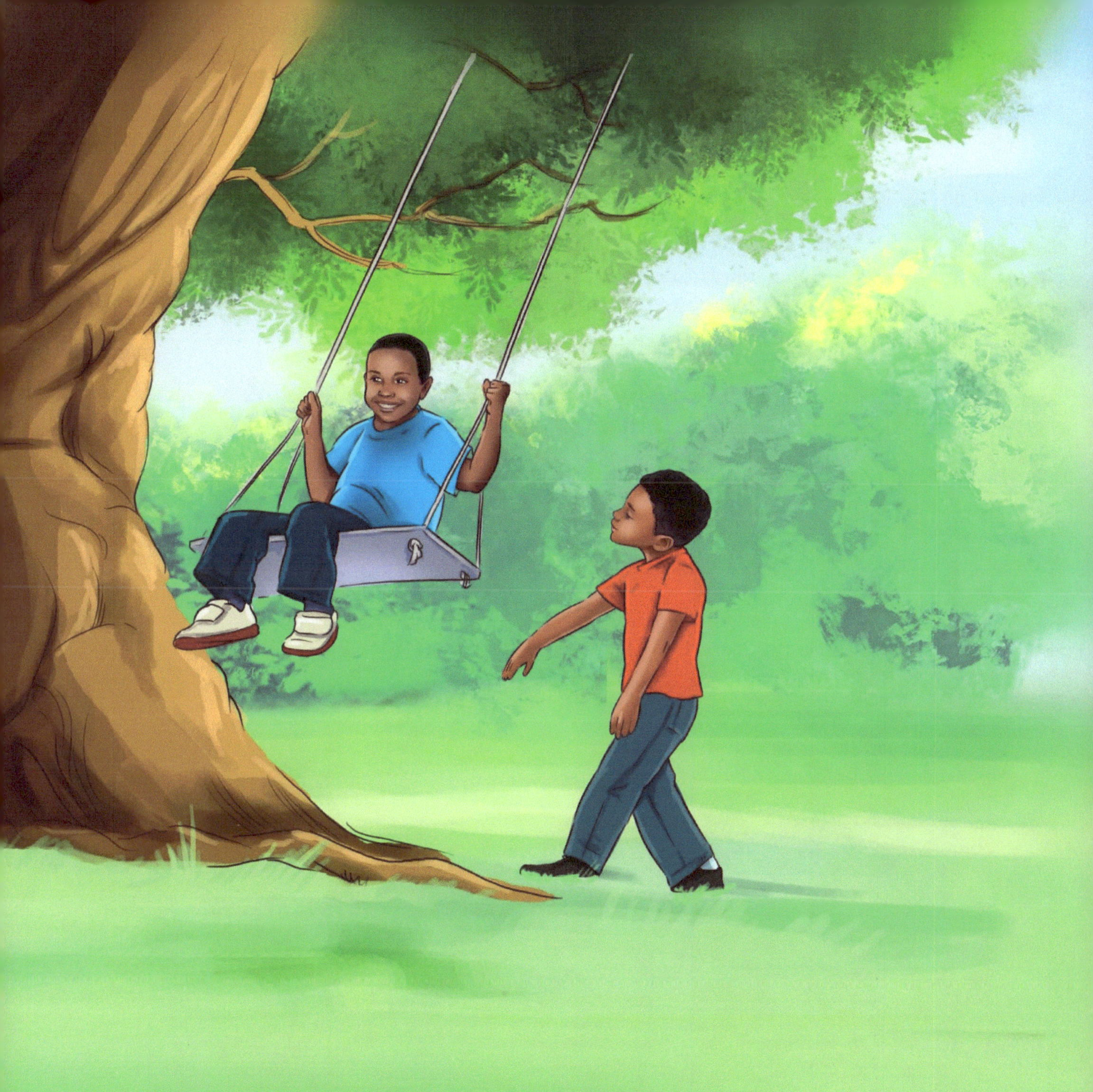

London replied, "Hambuggas please!"

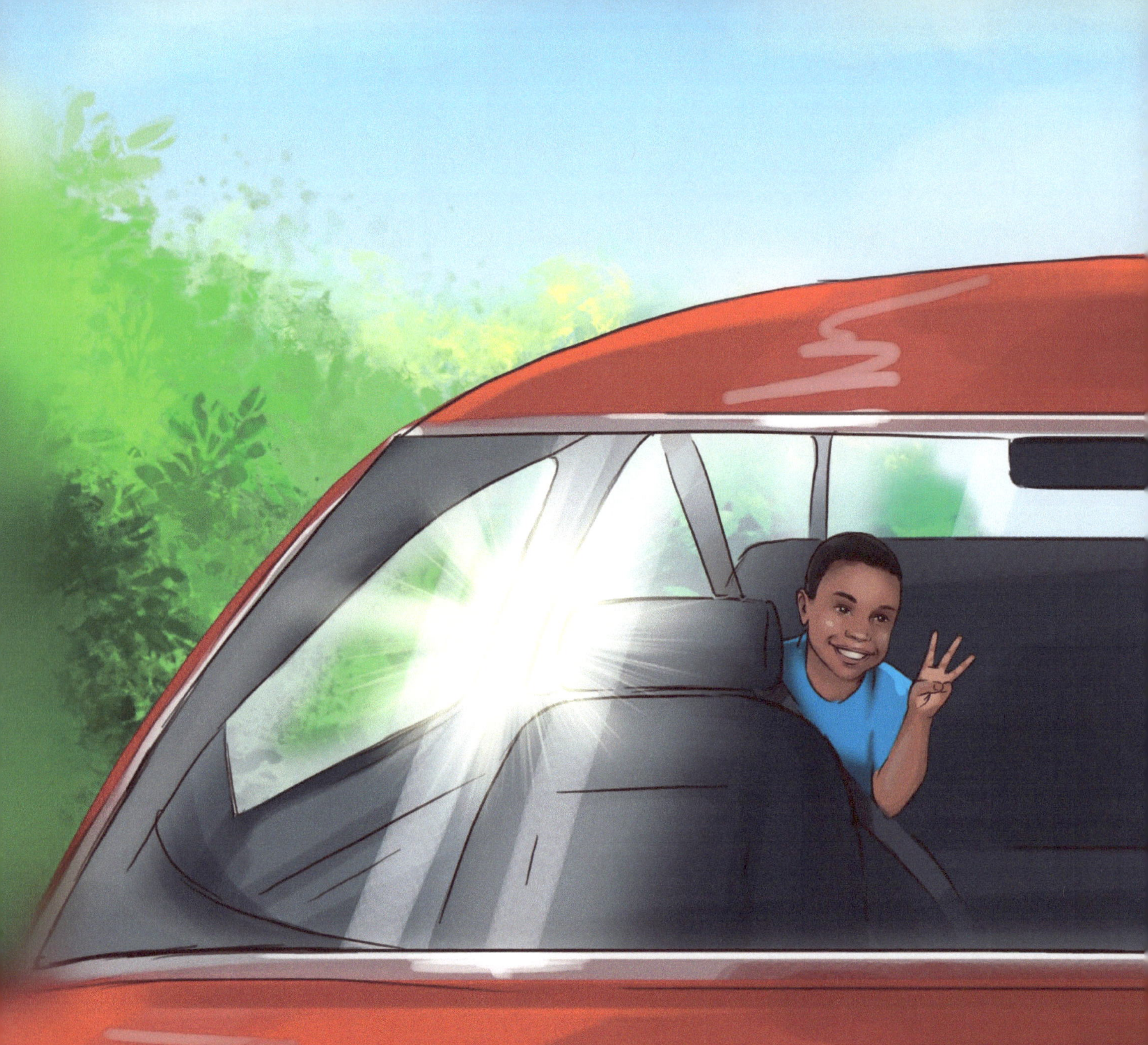

"Grandma G, I just love hambuggas. I love everybody's hambuggas. Can I have 3?"

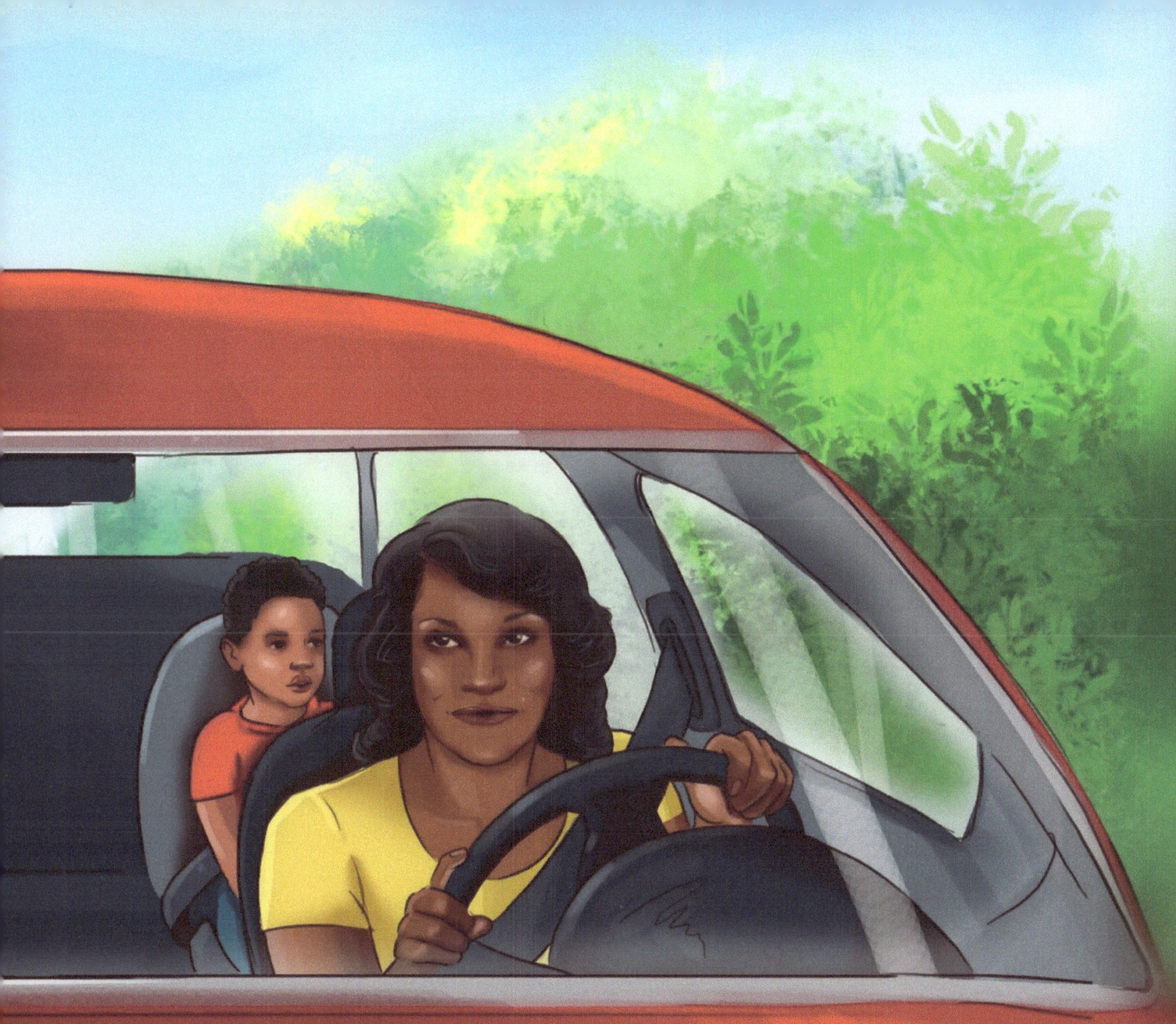

"Are you kidding me? That's too much bread. 1 big hamburger is all you need," said Grandma G.

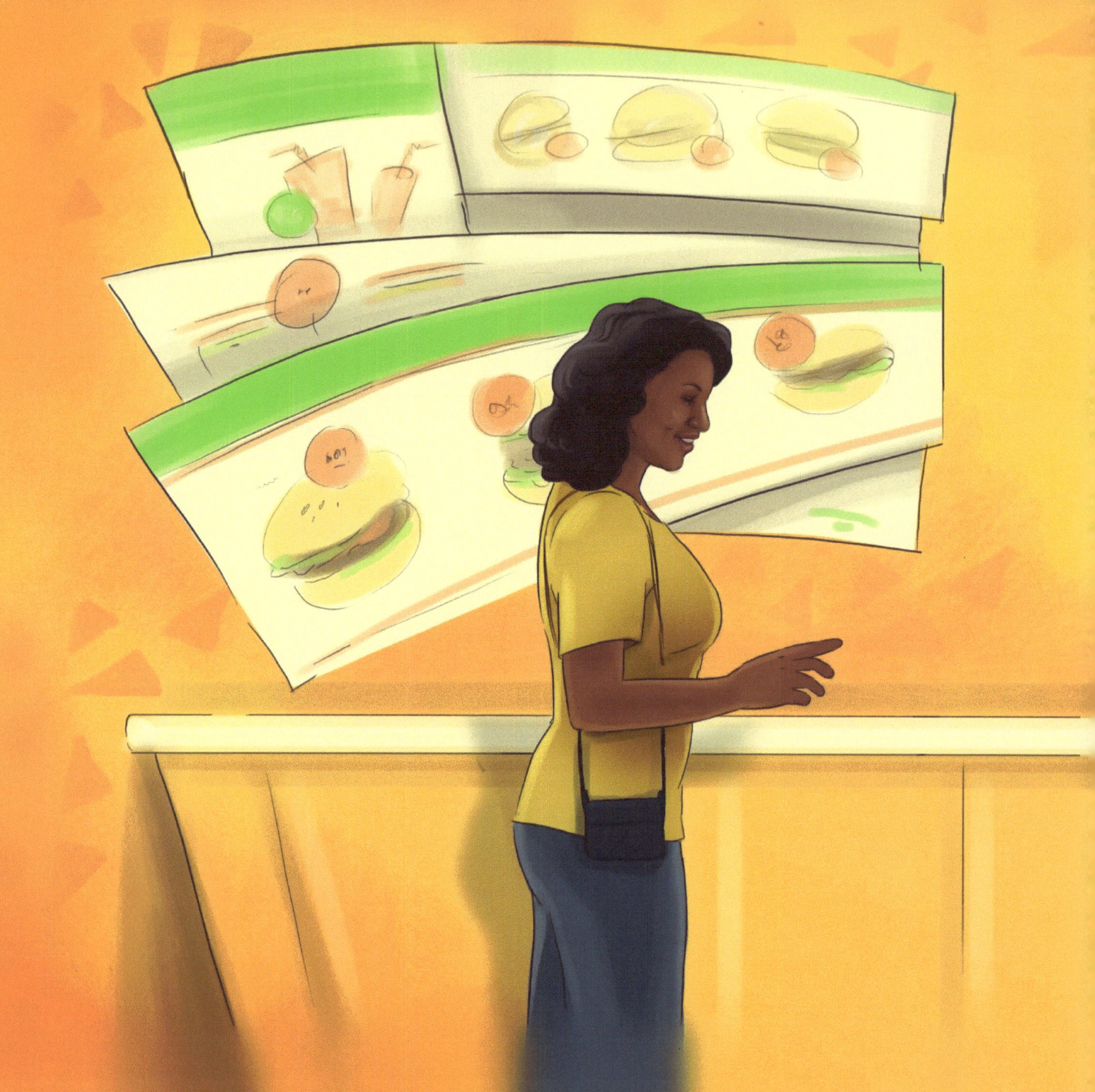

Grandma said, "The biggest burger
may be too big for your hands. Can
you eat it all? I'm not sure you can."

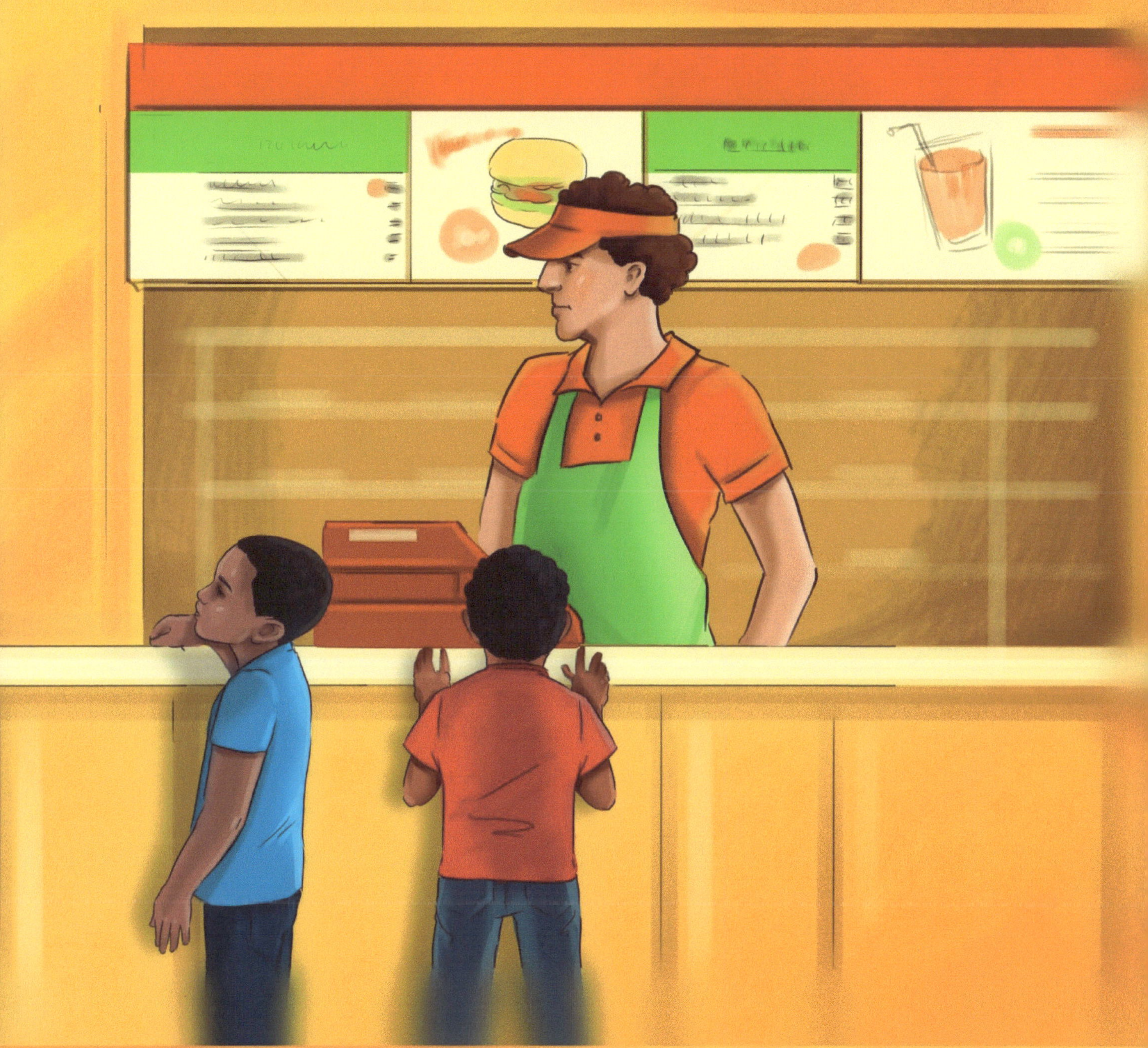

London said, " Grandma G,
I will eat it, I surely can.
That hambugga will fit in my hand."

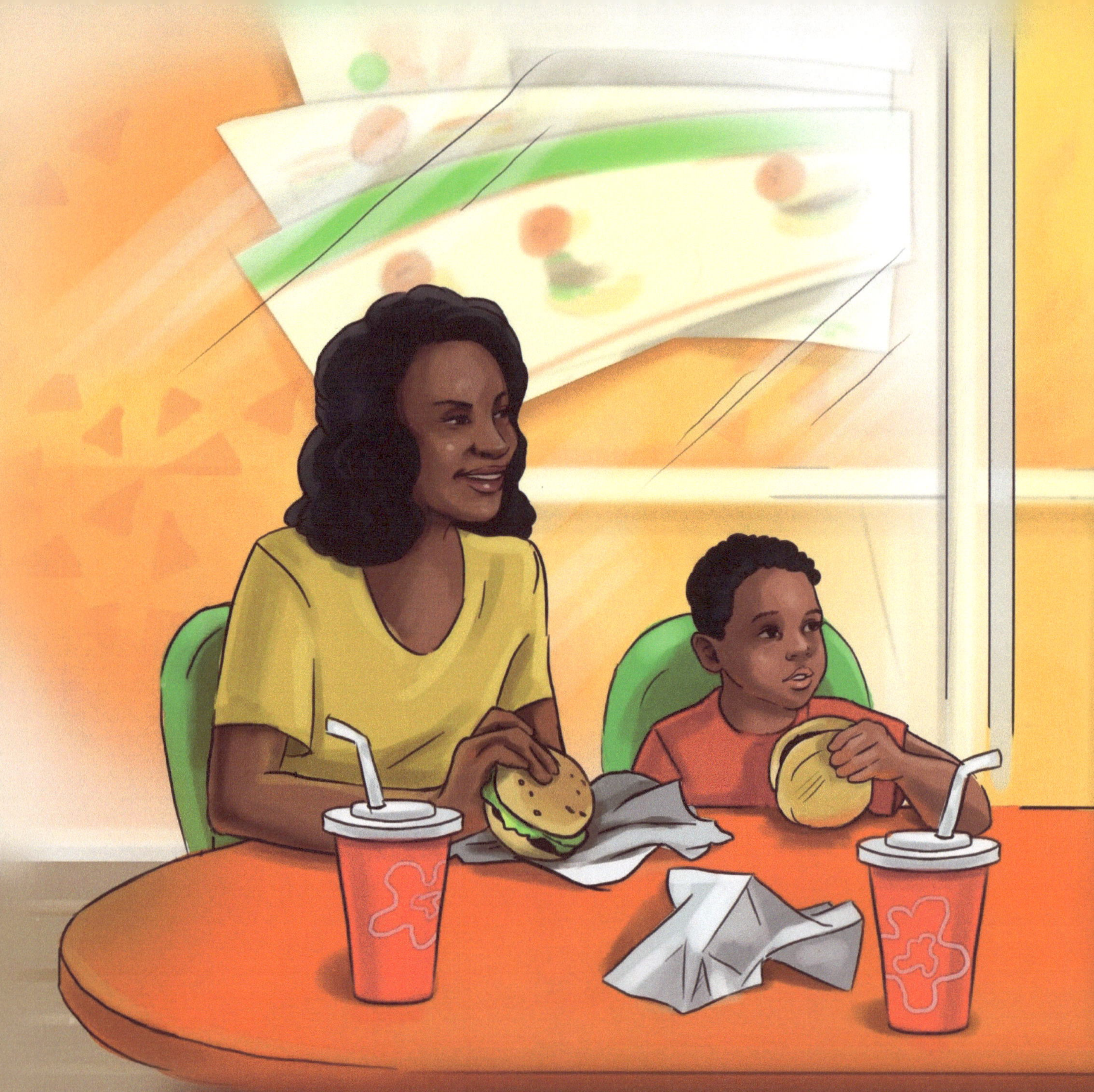

When London ate a hamburger, he
was elated. He was animated.

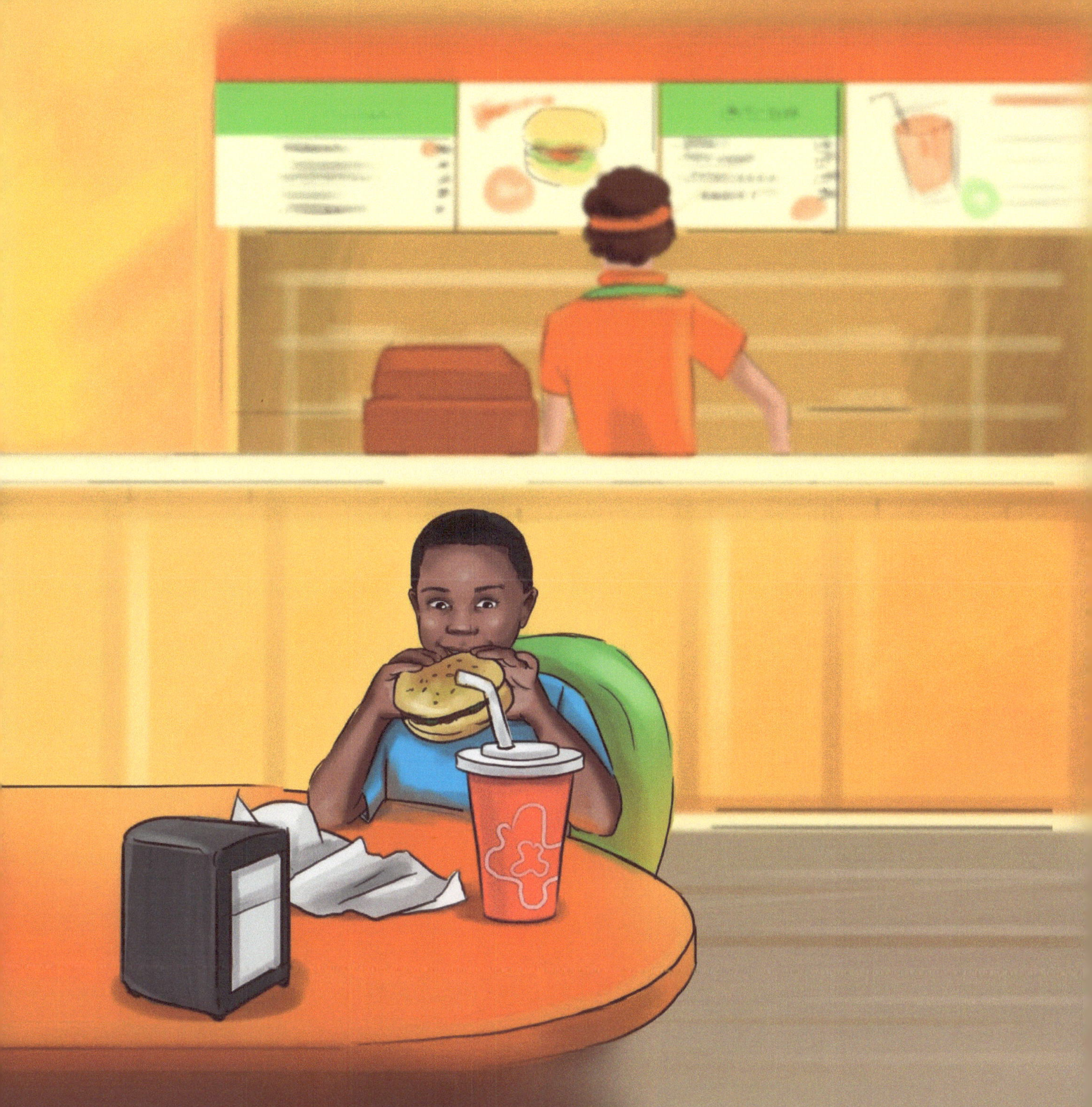

"Big eyes"
"Bright smile"
"Every time he ate um!"

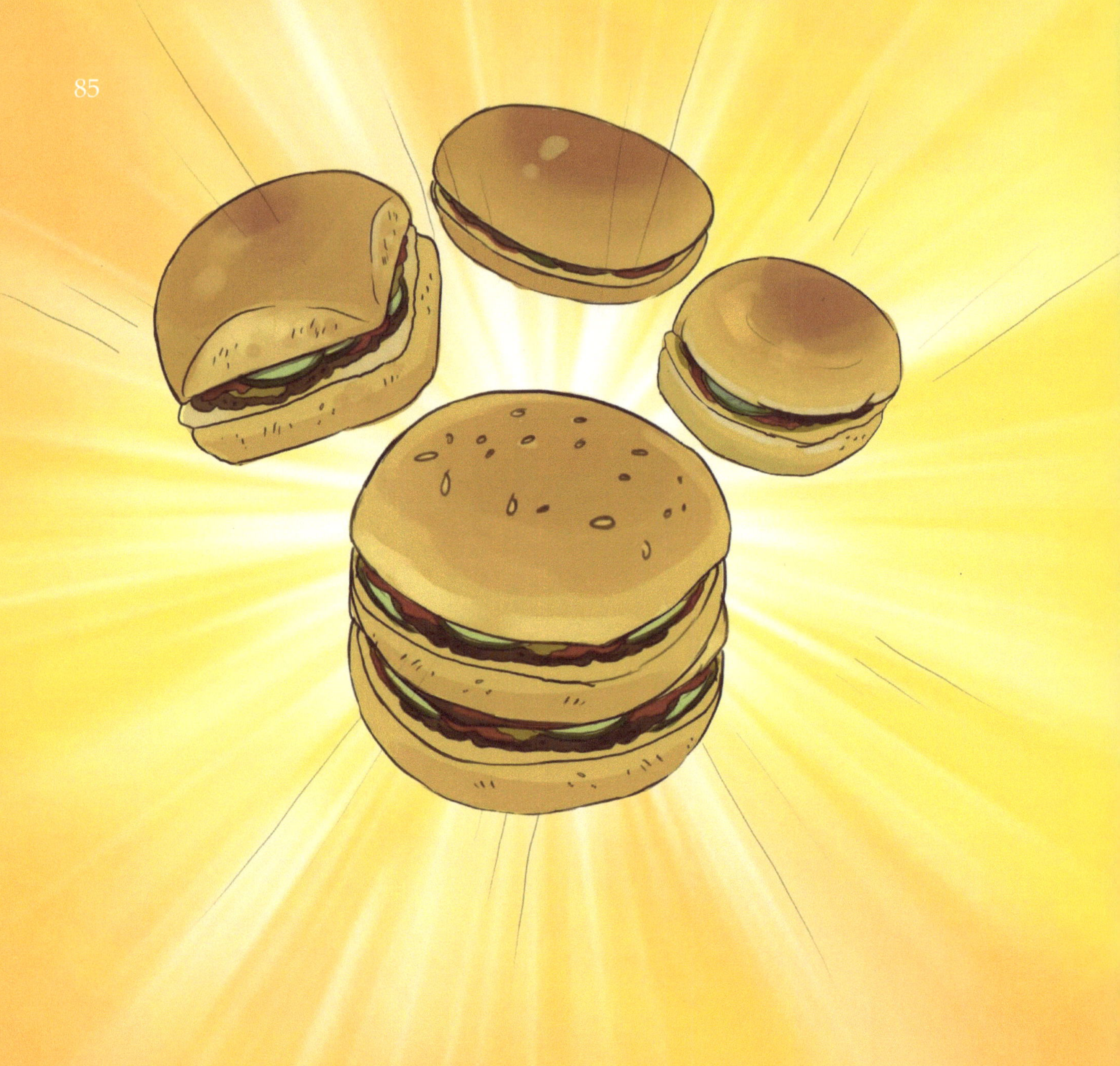

"London loved hamburgers, round or square, as long as it was a hamburger, he didn't care.

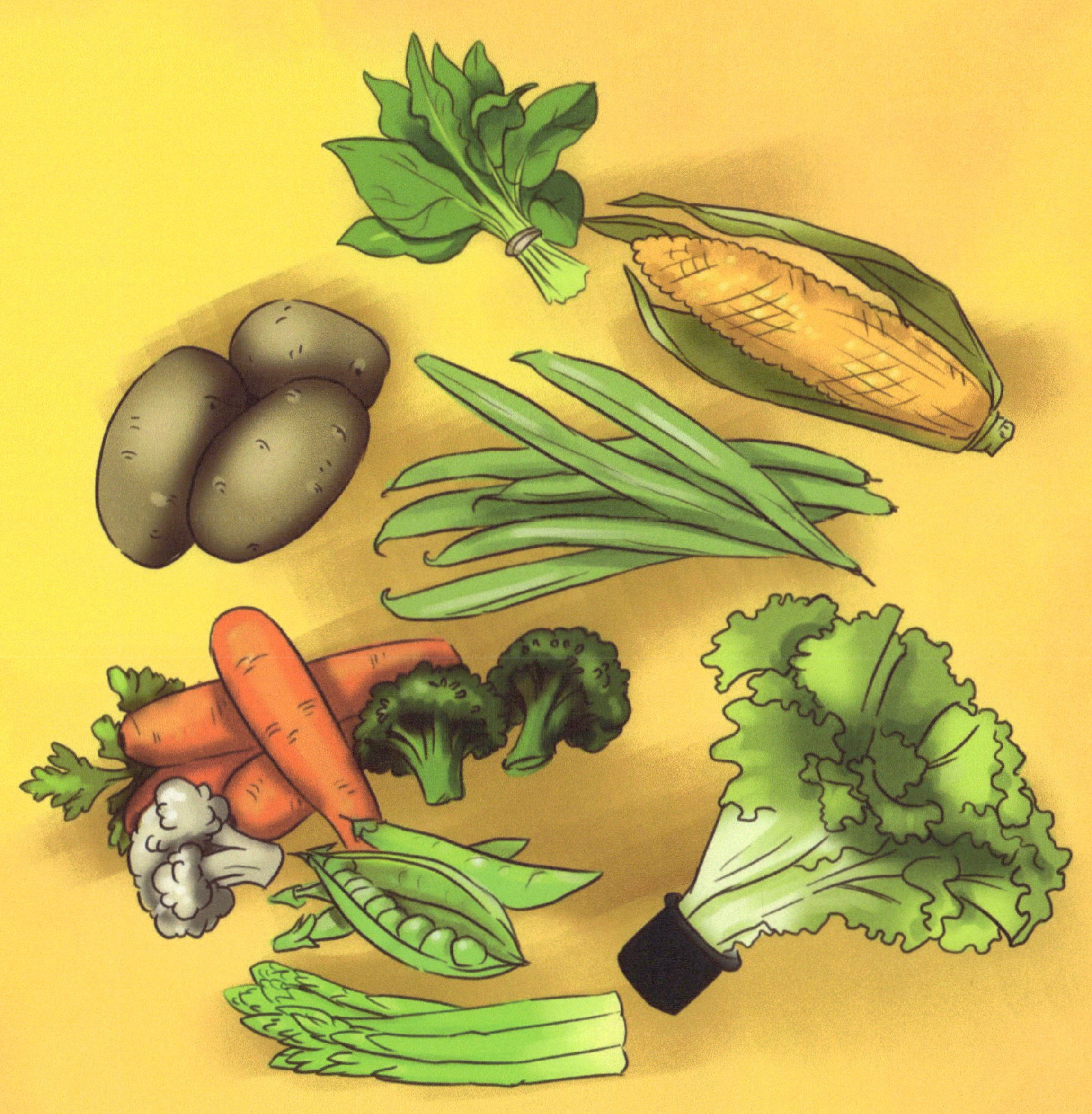

Thin or thick, big or small, but
he didn't like vegetables at all!

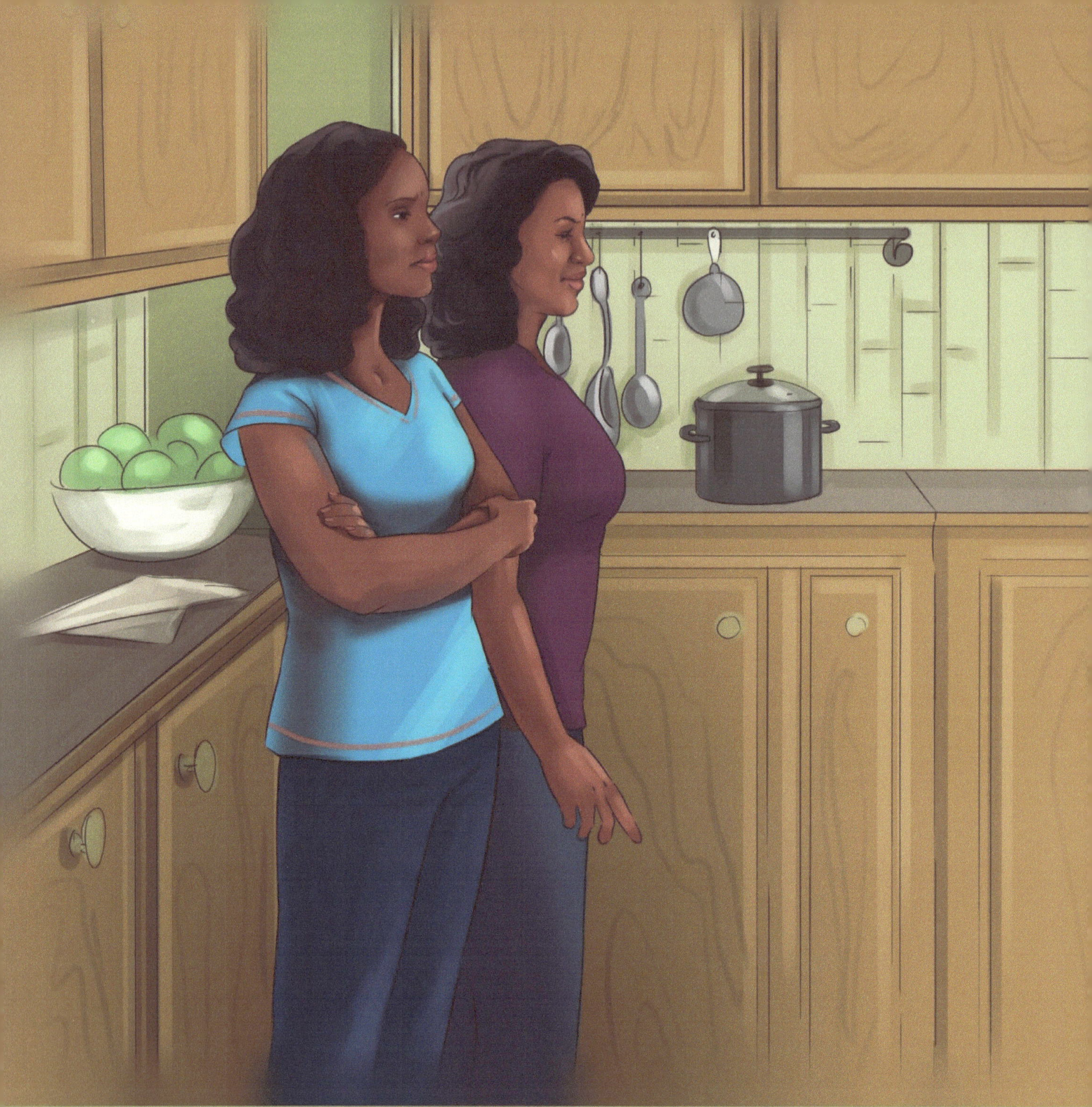

Mom insisted, "Eat your vegetables, London, Lourde you too. Vegetables are good for you."

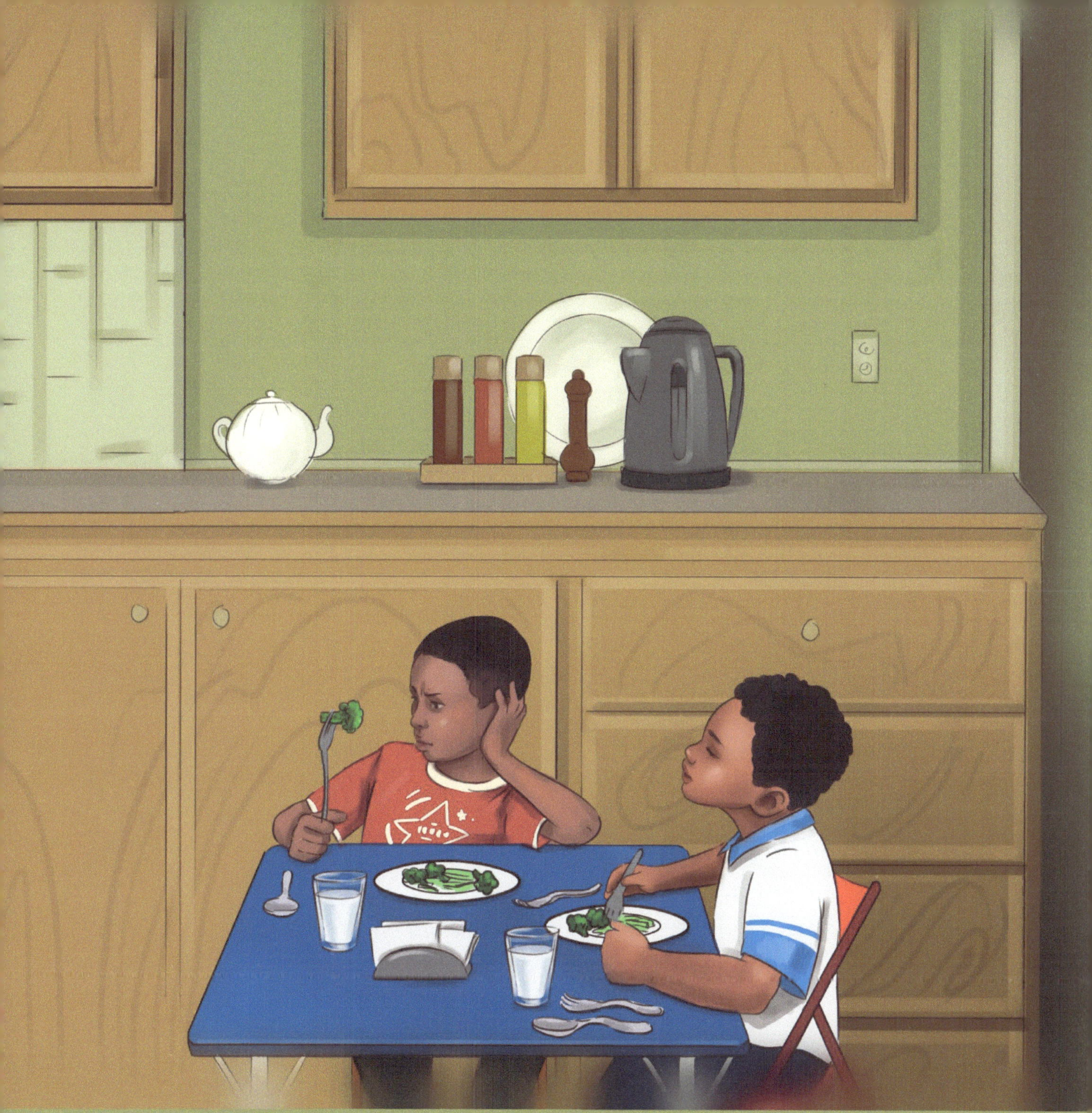

London stares at the broccoli
as if it's weird. What Mom
told him brings him to tears.

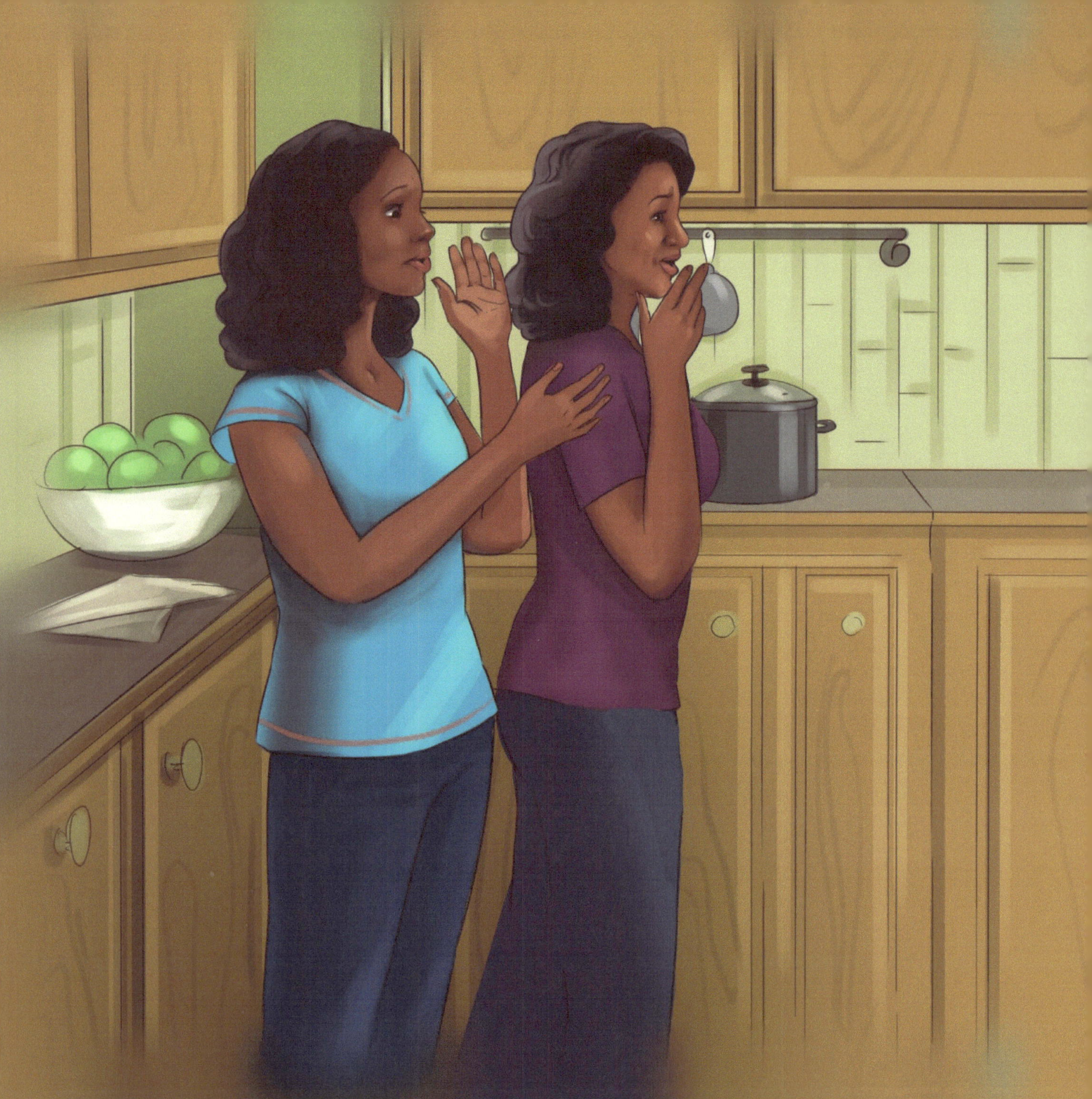

London covers his mouth; he gags
and frowns. For some strange
reason, the broccoli won't go down.

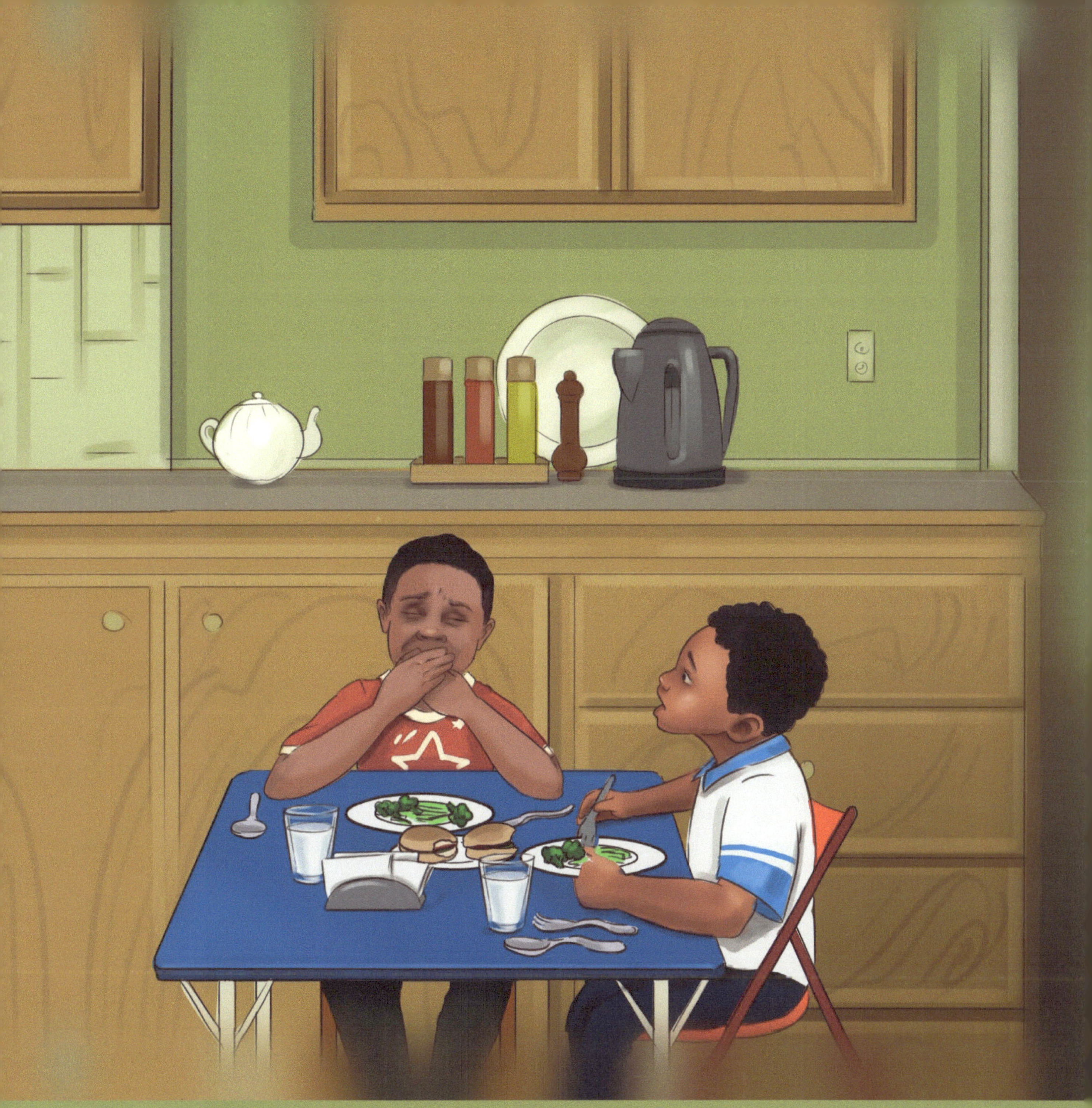

Mom and Grandma says, "OH NO!
UP CHUCK, UP CHUCK, he's going to blow!"

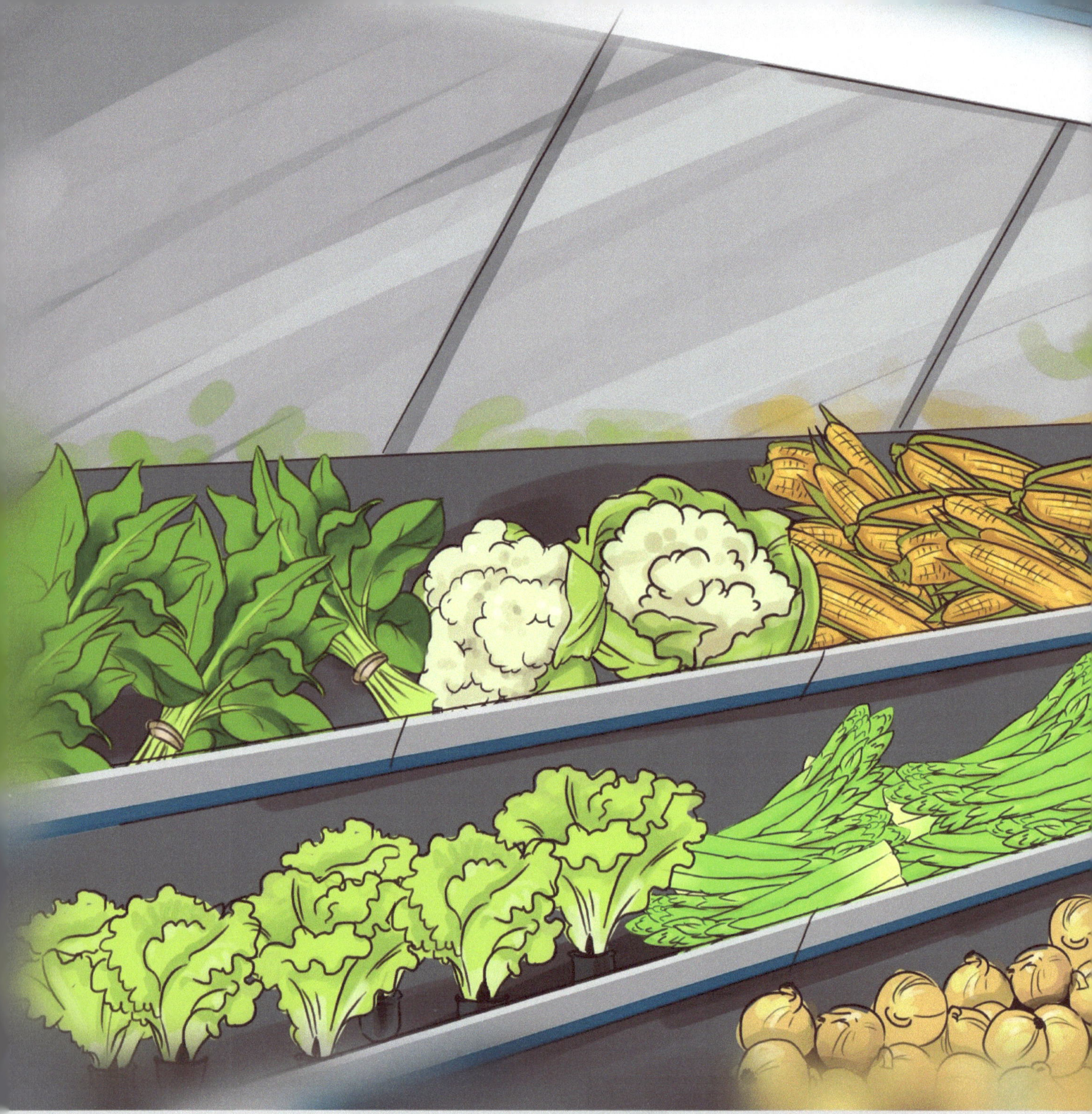

Grandma went to the store, she bought
peas, corn, asparagus, and more.

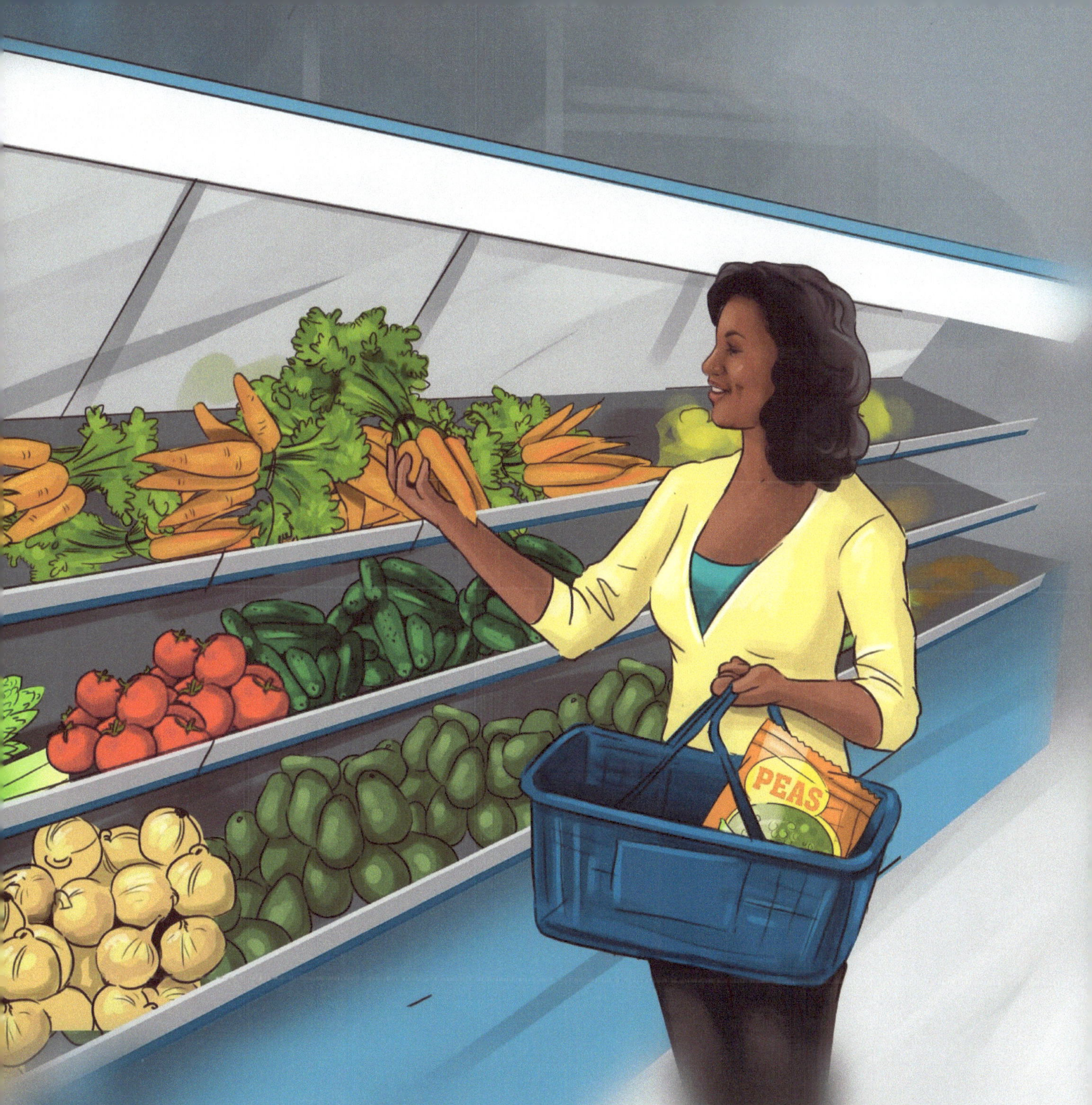

Vegetables London up chucked, what a great
feat, to find a vegetable London would eat.

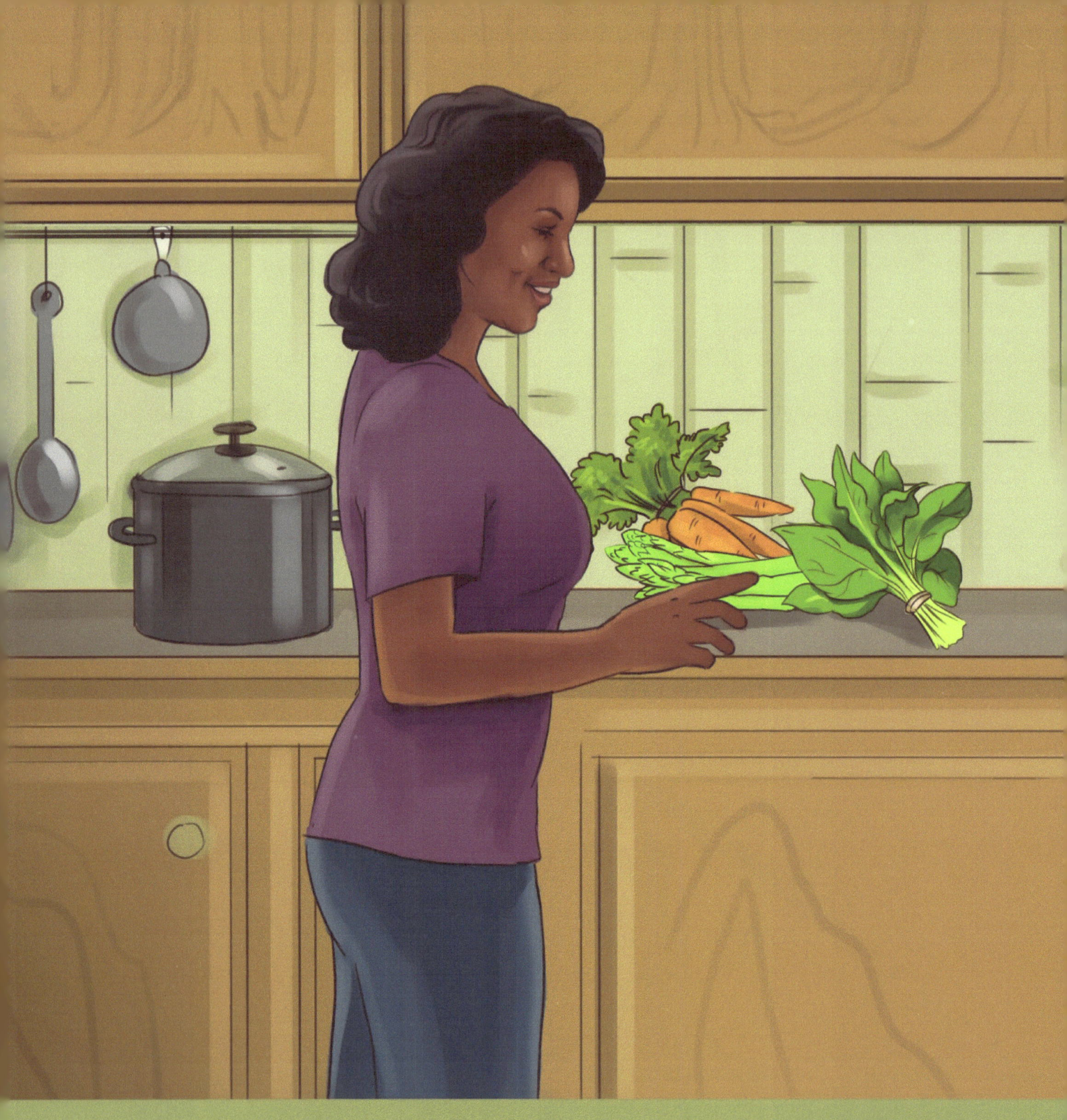

Grandma told London, "Vegetables give your body what it needs, to help keep you healthy so you can succeed."

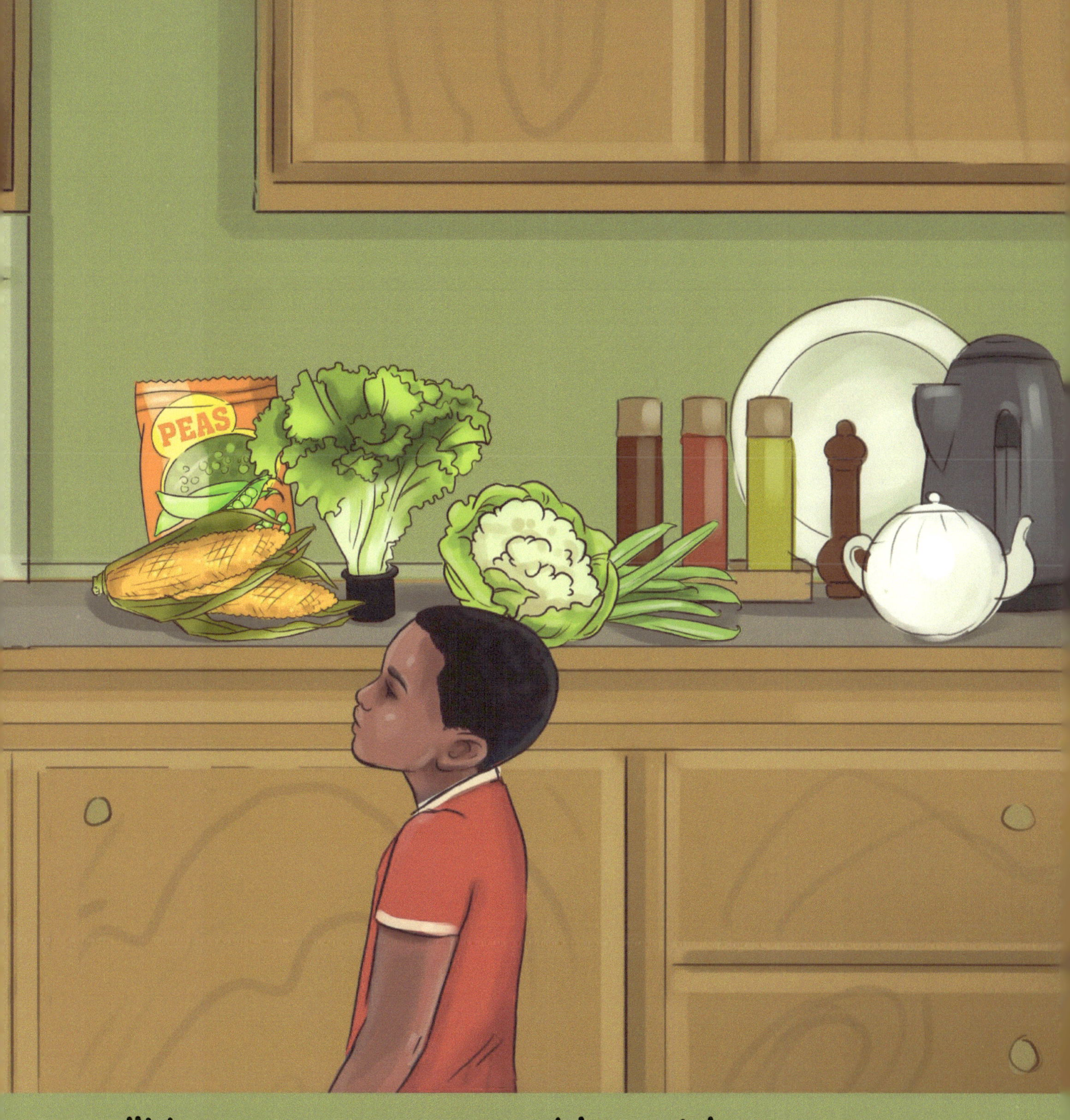

"Here are some vegetables, pick one you like, one you think would taste just right."

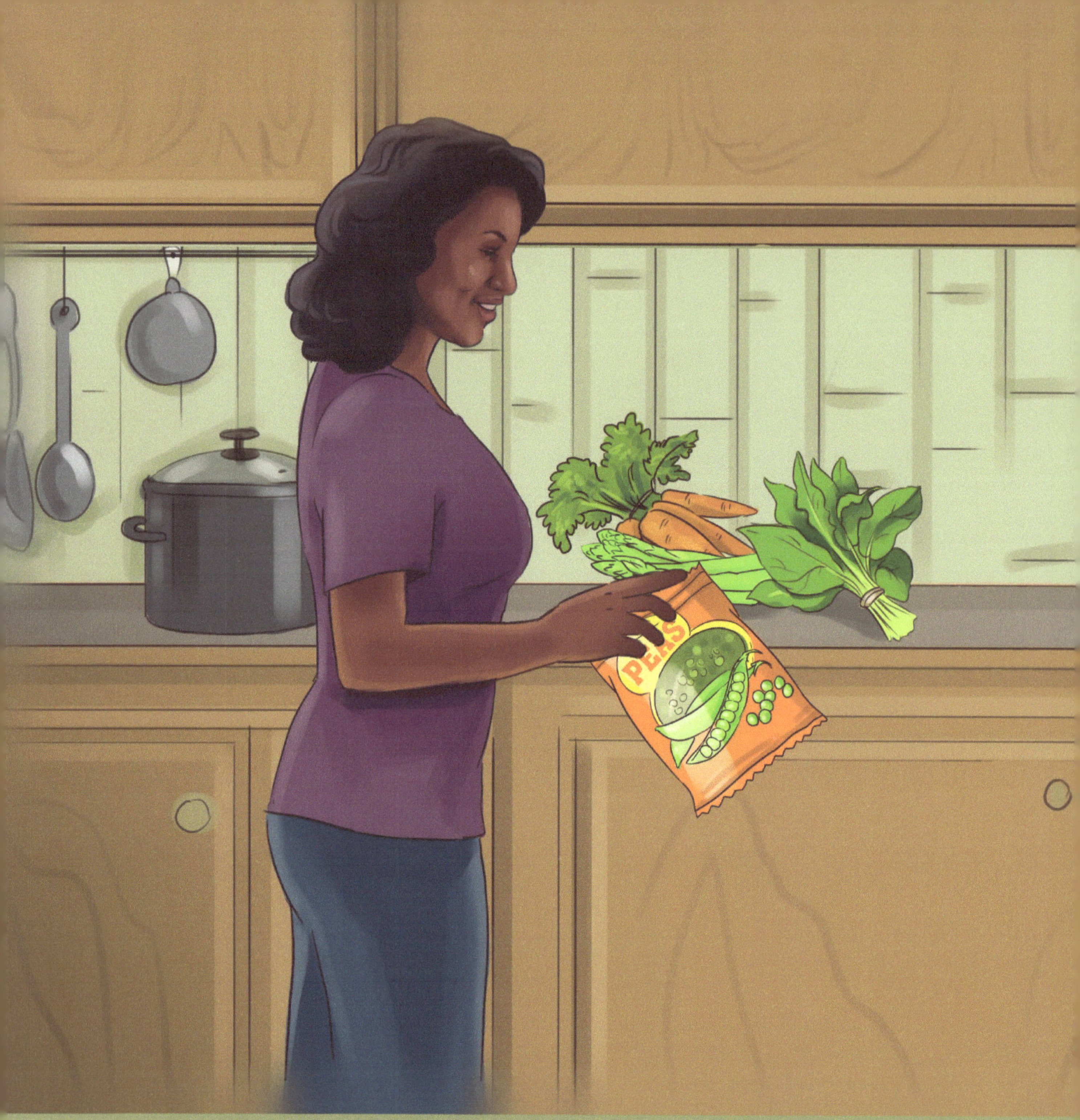

Frozen peas he did pick. He said
they wouldn't make him sick.

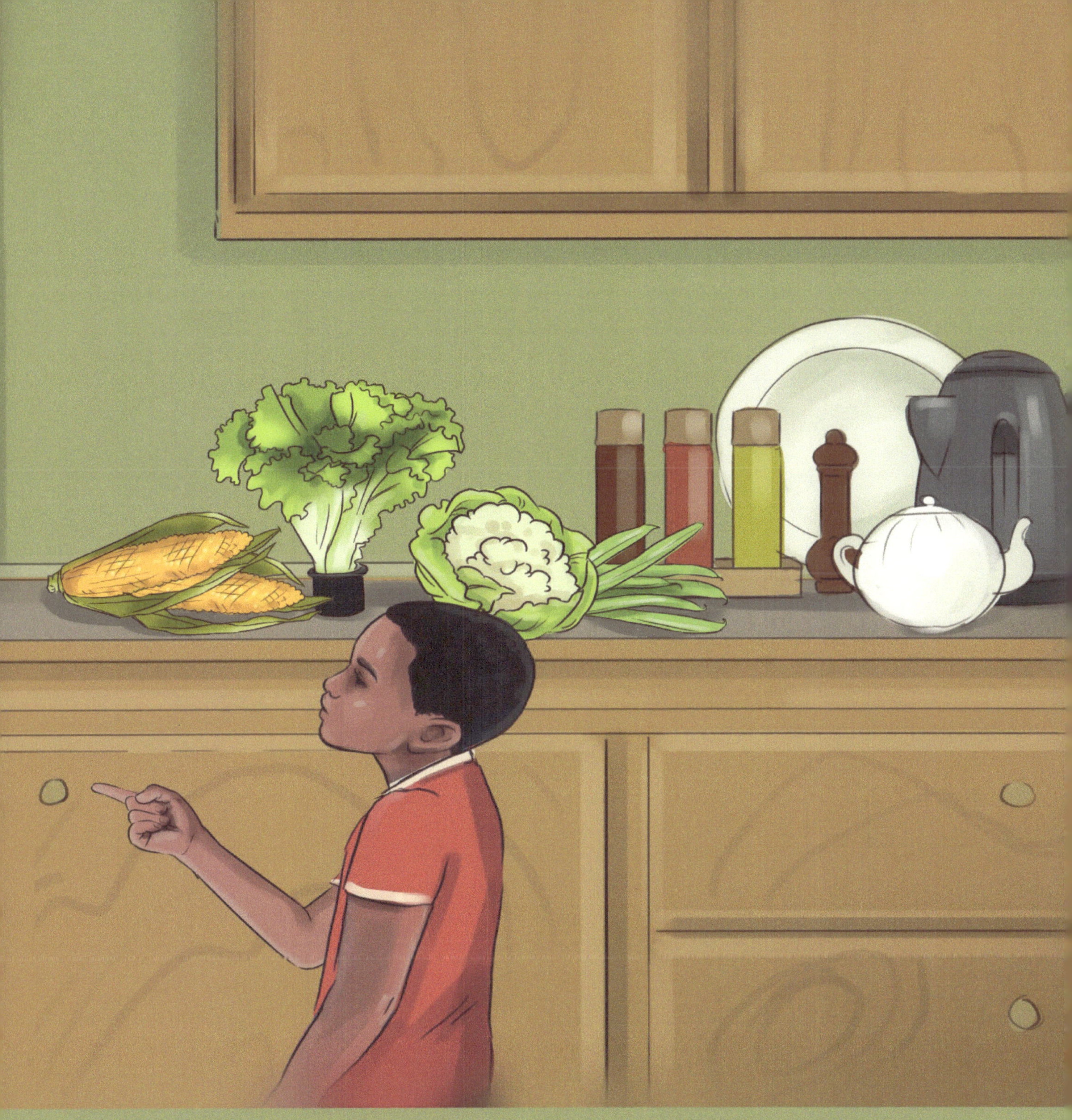

Grandma said, "That works for me, straight from the bag, they're ready to eat."

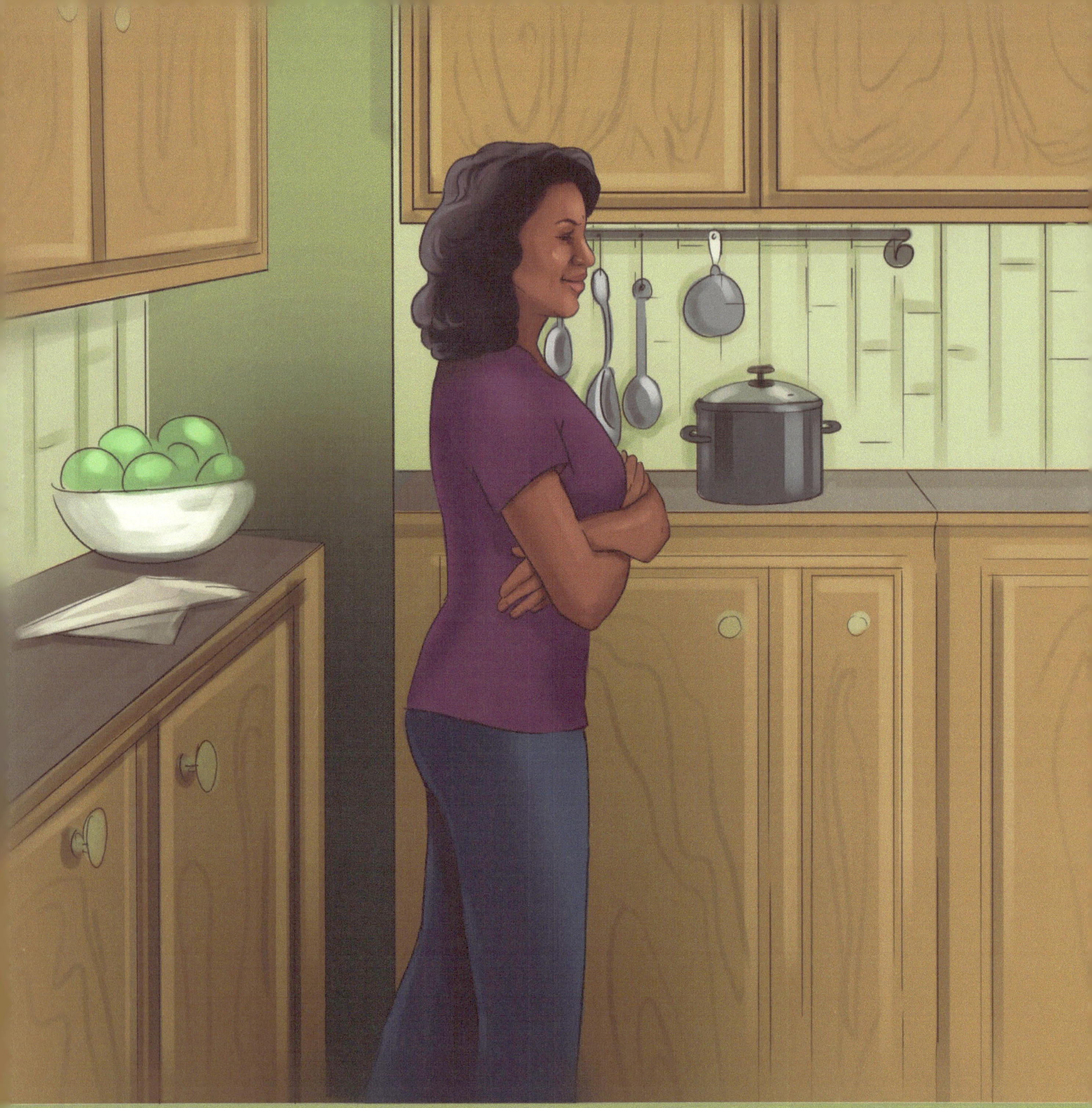

Small, round, green and sweet,
peas became a frequent treat.

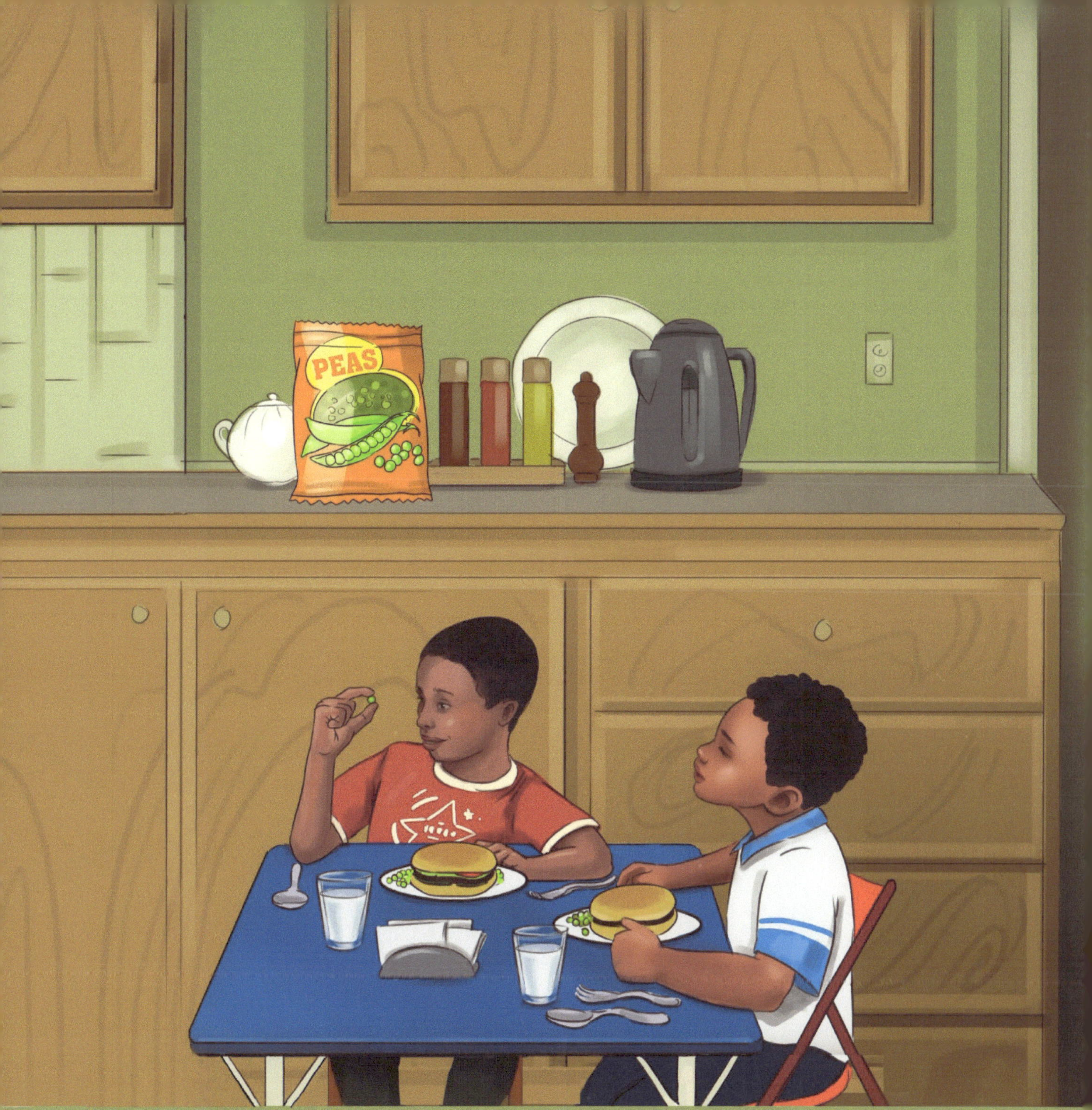

To his belly, peas went down.
Smiles, smiles, all around.

What about Lourde?
Well, he's alright.
He mostly ate what his
big brother liked.
Now, lettuce, tomato,
extra pickles, and cheese,
are on his hamburger
beside his peas. Now his
body has what it needs.

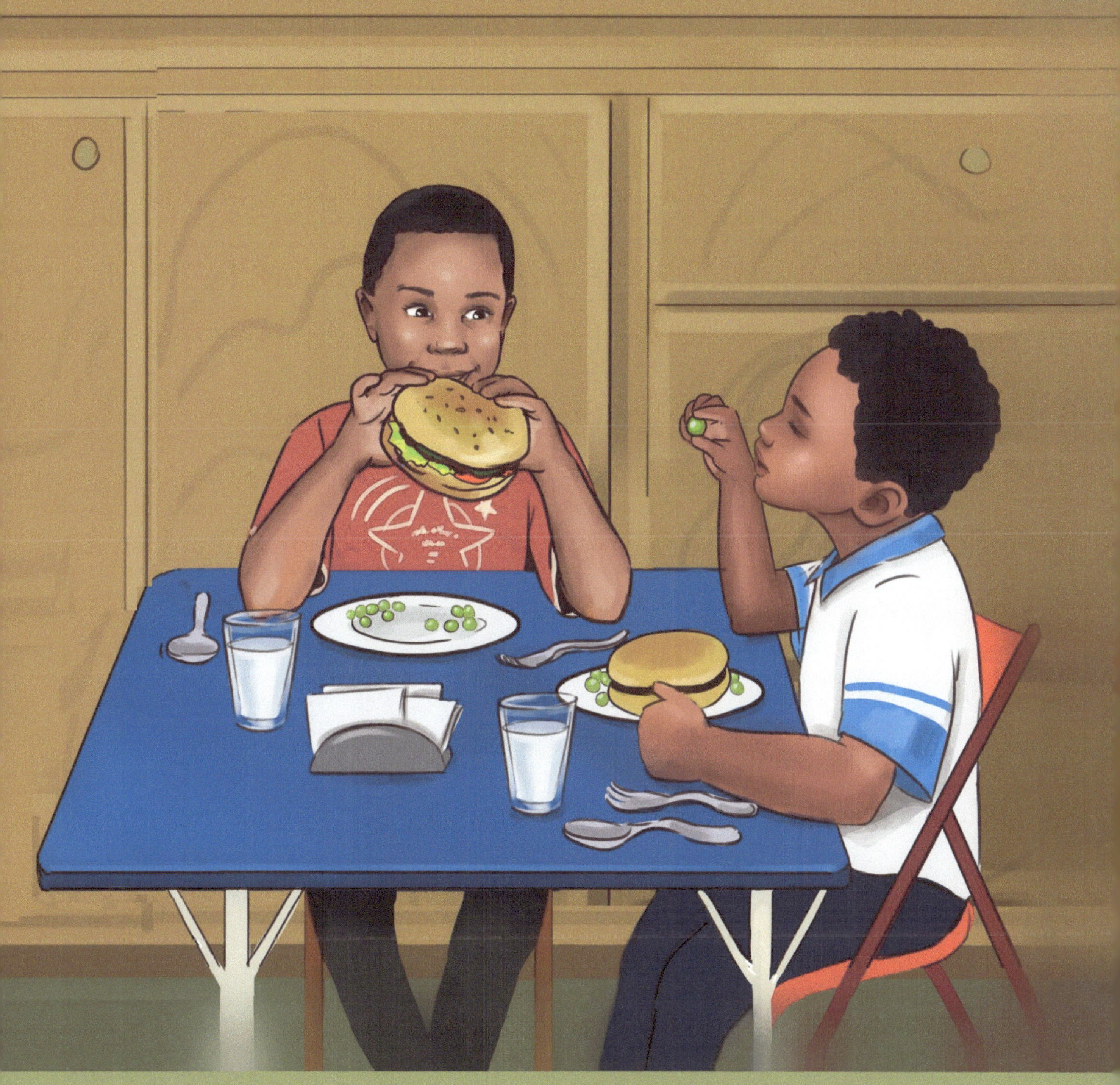

"Lourde agrees."
He likes the peas.

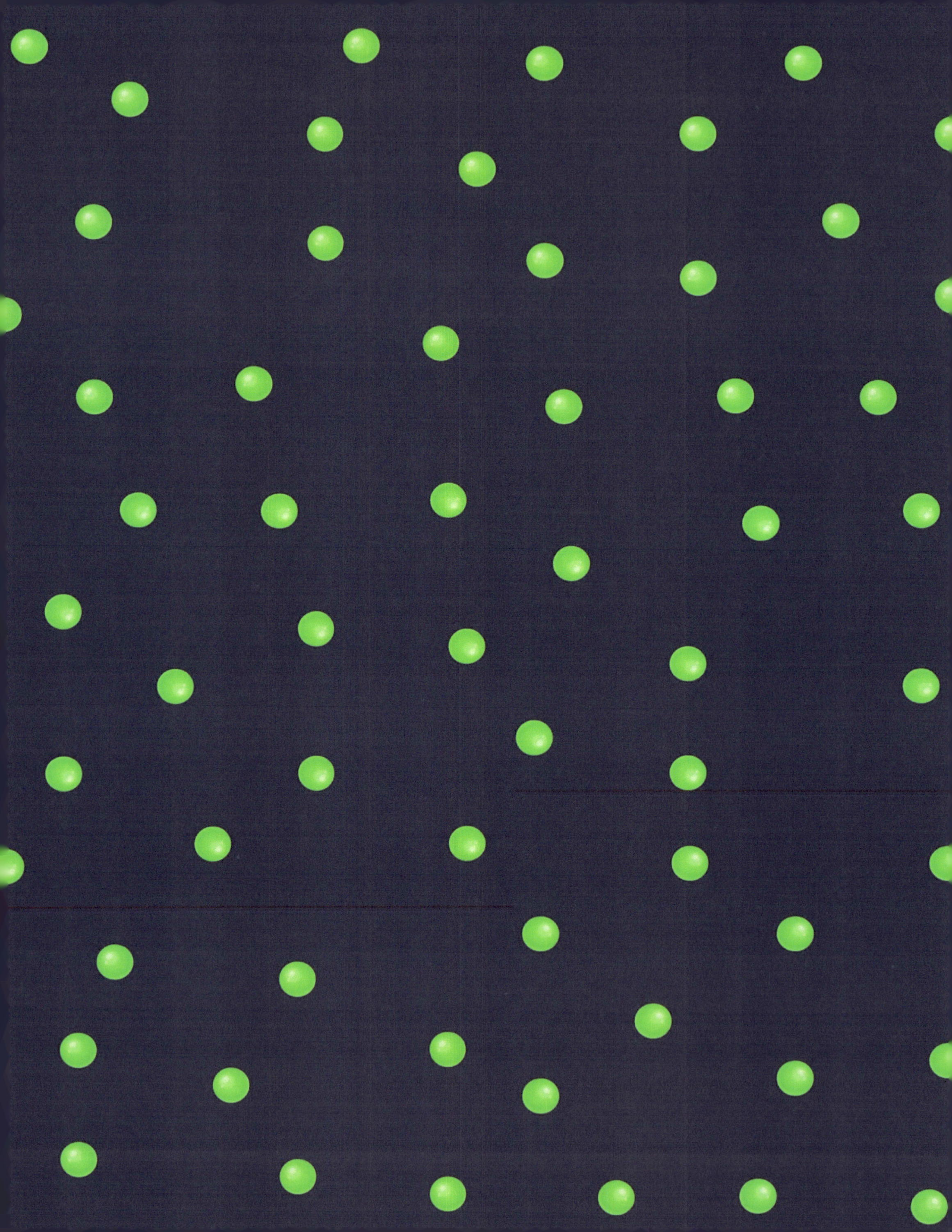

Frozen Peas

Frozen peas 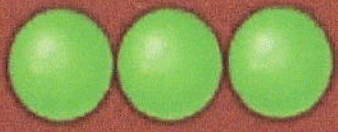 little circles round and green.

Frozen peas add one more, now the quantity is 4.

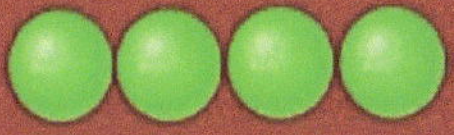

Frozen peas are very sweet. 5 can be a tasty treat.

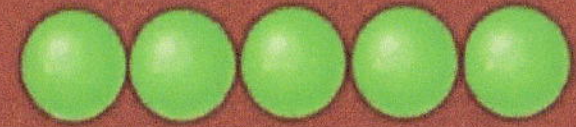

Frozen peas, "Peas rhyme with Bees."
How many bees do you see? 6

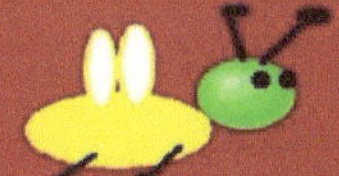  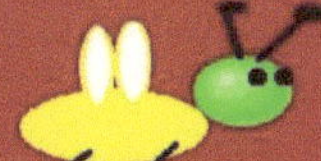 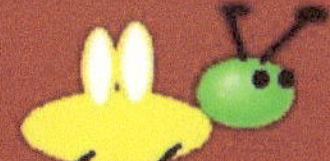  

Frozen peas can make more shapes,
when counting 7 and counting 8.

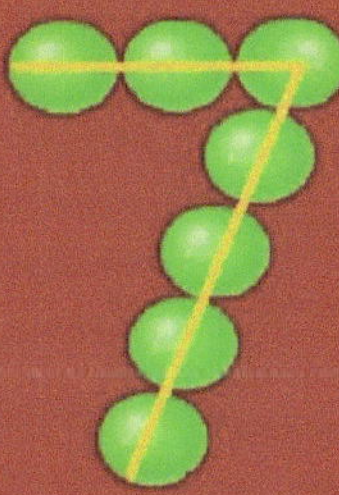 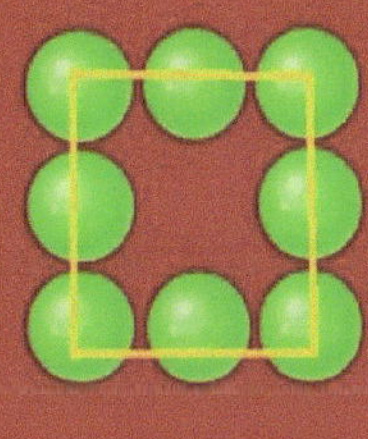

Frozen peas can make a line.
Lay them straight and count to 9.

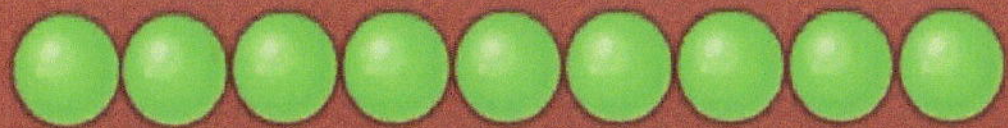

Frozen peas, count 1-10, then we can begin again.

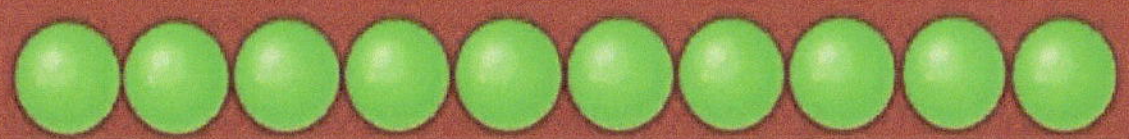